# The Vegan Power

## *120 Easy Vegan Recipes for Beginners*

# Introduction

I want to thank you and congratulate you for downloading the book, *"The Vegan Power: 120 Easy Vegan Recipes for Beginners"*.

This book offers 120 easy vegan recipes. It is a follow up to my first book **"The Vegan Power: Why Going Vegan Will Save Your Life"**.

It contains recipes that are easy to follow and fun to prepare. These recipes not only will help you improve your health but will also allow you to have more energy and focus better throughout the day. Being a vegan is not just about eating vegetables, there are thousands of things that can be eaten and this book will teach you how to use them while preparing your meals and how to cook them to perfection.

Thanks again for downloading this book, I hope you enjoy it!

information is without contract or any type of guarantee assurance.

The trademarks that are used are without any consent, and the publication of the trademark is without permission or backing by the trademark owner. All trademarks and brands within this book are for clarifying purposes only and are the owned by the owners themselves, not affiliated with this document.

# Contents

# Chapter 1

# 20 Breakfast Recipes

# Whole Wheat Pancakes

## Ingredients

- 1 cup whole wheat flour
- 2/3 cup all-purpose flour
- 1/3 cup wheat germ
- 1 1/2 teaspoons baking powder
- 1/2 teaspoon baking soda
- 2 tablespoons brown sugar
- 1 teaspoon salt
- 5 1/3 tablespoons unsalted butter
- 2 1/2 cups buttermilk
- 2 eggs, beaten
- 3 tablespoons unsalted butter

## Instructions

1. In a food processor or in a large bowl, combine the whole wheat flour, white flour, wheat germ or oats, baking powder, baking soda, brown sugar, and salt
2. Cut the butter into small pieces with a knife, and add the butter to the flour-mixture. Mix until the mixture has a sand-like consistency
3. Make a well in the center of the flour-butter mixture, and add the buttermilk and eggs. Stir until the liquids are fully incorporated
4. Heat a frying pan over medium heat and grease the surface with 1 tablespoon of butter or oil. Ladle the

batter onto the surface to form 4 inch pancakes. Once bubbles form on the top of the pancakes, flip them over, and cook them on the other side for about 2 minutes

# Tofu Quiche with Broccoli

Ingredients

- 1 (9 inch) unbaked 9 inch pie crust
- 1 pound broccoli, chopped
- 1 tablespoon olive oil
- 1 onion, finely chopped
- 4 cloves garlic, minced
- 1 pound firm tofu, drained
- 1/2 cup soy milk
- 1/4 teaspoon Dijon mustard
- 3/4 teaspoon salt
- 1/4 teaspoon ground nutmeg
- 1/2 teaspoon ground red pepper
- black pepper to taste
- 1 tablespoon dried parsley
- 1/8 cup Parmesan flavor soy cheese

Instructions

1. Preheat oven to 400 degrees F (200 degrees C). Bake pie crust in preheated oven for 10 to 12 minutes.
2. Place broccoli in a steamer over 1 inch of boiling water, and cover. Cook until tender but still firm, about 2 to 6 minutes. Drain.
3. Heat oil in a large skillet over medium-high heat. Sauté onion and garlic until golden. Stir in the cooked broccoli and heat through.

4. In a blender, combine tofu, soy milk, mustard, salt, nutmeg, ground red pepper, black pepper, parsley and Parmesan soy cheese; process until smooth. In a large bowl combine tofu mixture with broccoli mixture. Pour into pie crust.
5. Bake in preheated oven until quiche is set, 35 to 40 minutes. Allow to stand for at least 5 minutes before cutting.

# Black Bean Breakfast Bowl

Ingredients

- 2 tablespoons olive oil
- 4 eggs, beaten
- 1 (15 ounce) can black beans, drained and rinsed
- 1 avocado, peeled and sliced
- 1/4 cup salsa
- salt and ground black pepper to taste

Instructions

1. Heat olive oil in a small pan over medium heat. Cook and stir eggs until eggs are set, 3 to 5 minutes.
2. Place black beans in a microwave-safe bowl. Heat on High in the microwave until warm, about 1 minute.
3. Divide warmed black beans between two bowls.
4. Top each bowl with scrambled eggs, avocado, and salsa. Season with salt and black pepper.

# Sweet Potato Breakfast Casserole

Ingredients

- 1 (8 ounce) package vegetarian sausage
- 1/2 cup water, or more as needed
- 4 cups shredded sweet potatoes
- 1/4 cup butter, melted
- 1 1/2 (8 ounce) packages shredded, reduced-fat mild Cheddar-mozzarella cheese blend
- 1/2 cup finely chopped onion
- 1 cup finely sliced fresh spinach leaves
- 1 (16 ounce) container low-fat small curd cottage cheese
- 8 jumbo eggs

Instructions

1. Preheat oven to 375 degrees F (190 degrees C). Lightly grease a 9x13-inch baking dish.
2. Place sausage in a large skillet and pour in about 1/4 inch of water; cook sausage over medium heat until water evaporates and sausages are evenly browned, 10 to 15 minutes. Crumble cooked sausages into a bowl.
3. Mix sweet potatoes and butter together in a bowl; evenly spread into the bottom of the prepared 9x13-inch dish.
4. Stir Cheddar-mozzarella cheese blend, onion, spinach, cottage cheese, eggs, and crumbled sausage together in a large bowl; spoon over sweet potato layer.

5.  Bake casserole in the preheated oven until a toothpick inserted in the center comes out clean and eggs are set, about 1 hour. Cool 5 minutes before serving.

# Easy Gorgonzola Tofu Scramble

Ingredients

- 1 1/2 tablespoons olive oil
- 1/3 (12 ounce) package extra-firm tofu, cut into cubes
- 1/4 cup chopped red onion
- 1 clove garlic, minced
- 2/3 cup sliced white mushrooms
- 1 cup packed fresh spinach
- 3 tablespoons crumbled Gorgonzola cheese

Instructions

1. Heat olive oil in a skillet over medium heat; cook and stir tofu, onion, and garlic until onion is translucent, 5 to 10 minutes. Add mushrooms; cook and stir until mushrooms are tender and tofu is lightly browned, 5 to 10 minutes.
2. Remove skillet from heat. Mix spinach and Gorgonzola cheese into tofu mixture until spinach begins to wilt and the cheese melts from the heat of the tofu mixture.

# Creamy Blueberry Coconut Ricotta Bowl

Ingredients

- 1/4 cup whole milk ricotta cheese
- 1 tablespoon coconut milk
- 1 tablespoon honey, or to taste
- 1 tablespoon slivered almond
- 1 tablespoon sweetened flaked coconut
- 1/2 cup blueberries, or to taste

Instructions

1. Combine ricotta cheese and coconut milk in a bowl. Drizzle on honey and sprinkle with almonds and coconut. Top with blueberries.

# Baked Granola Bars

Ingredients

- 3/4 cup grounded oats
- 1 cup water
- 3/4 cup dates
- 1/2 cup chia seeds
- 1/4 cup sunflower seeds
- 1/4 cup pumpkin seeds
- 1/4 cup dried cranberries (chopped)
- 1 teaspoon cinnamon
- 1 teaspoon vanilla extract
- 1/4 teaspoon salt

Instructions

1. Preheat oven to 325 F
2. Set up a pan with a piece of over paper
3. Blend the rolled oats and then put it in a large bowl
4. Blend the dates with the water
5. Add the dates and water mix to the large bowl and stir until combined with the rolled oats flour
6. Spread the mixture into the pan
7. Bake it for 25 minutes
8. Let it cool down for 10 minute
9. Slice and enjoy!

# Crustless Spinach Quiche

Ingredients

- 1 tablespoon vegetable oil
- 1 onion, chopped
- 1 (10 ounce) package frozen chopped spinach, thawed and drained
- 5 eggs, beaten
- 3 cups shredded Muenster cheese
- 1/4 teaspoon salt
- 1/8 teaspoon ground black pepper

Instructions

1. Preheat oven to 350 degrees F (175 degrees C). Lightly grease a 9 inch pie pan.
2. Heat oil in a large skillet over medium-high heat. Add onions and cook, stirring occasionally, until onions are soft. Stir in spinach and continue cooking until excess moisture has evaporated.
3. In a large bowl, combine eggs, cheese, salt and pepper. Add spinach mixture and stir to blend. Scoop into prepared pie pan.
4. Bake in preheated oven until eggs have set, about 30 minutes. Let cool for 10 minutes before serving.

# Fluffy Pancakes

Ingredients

- 3/4 cup milk
- 2 tablespoons white vinegar
- 1 cup all-purpose flour
- 2 tablespoons white sugar
- 1 teaspoon baking powder
- 1/2 teaspoon baking soda
- 1/2 teaspoon salt
- 1 egg
- 2 tablespoons butter, melted
- cooking spray

Instructions

1. Combine milk with vinegar in a medium bowl and set aside for 5 minutes to "sour".
2. Combine flour, sugar, baking powder, baking soda, and salt in a large mixing bowl. Whisk egg and butter into "soured" milk. Pour the flour mixture into the wet ingredients and whisk until lumps are gone.
3. Heat a large skillet over medium heat, and coat with cooking spray. Pour 1/4 cupfuls of batter onto the skillet, and cook until bubbles appear on the surface. Flip with a spatula, and cook until browned on the other side.

# Nutty Cinnamon Quinoa

Ingredients

- 1 cup vegan milk
- 1 cup water
- 1 cup rinsed quinoa
- 2 cups fresh blackberries
- 1/2 teaspoon ground cinnamon
- 1/3 cup toasted pecans (chopped)
- 4 teaspoons agave

Instructions

1. Boil water, vegan milk and quinoa in a saucepan on low heat for 10/15 minutes until liquid part is absorbed
2. Let rest for 10 minutes
3. Put the quinoa into a bowl
4. Add pecans, blackberries and agave

# Egg in a Boat

Ingredients

- 1/2 tablespoon butter
- 1 slice white bread
- 1 egg

Instructions

1. Butter both sides of bread. Cut a circular hole in the center of the slice of bread, about 2 1/2 inches in diameter.
2. Heat a frying pan or griddle on medium-high heat. When the frying pan is hot, place the bread into the pan and let it brown for one minute. Flip the toast over and let the other side brown for one minute.
3. Break the egg into the hole in the bread. Cook for 2 minutes, or until the egg is cooked to the consistency you prefer.

# Easy Broccoli Quiche

Ingredients

- 2 tablespoons butter
- 1 onion, minced
- 1 teaspoon minced garlic
- 2 cups chopped fresh broccoli
- 1 (9 inch) unbaked pie crust
- 1 1/2 cups shredded mozzarella cheese
- 4 eggs, well beaten
- 1 1/2 cups milk
- 1 teaspoon salt
- 1/2 teaspoon black pepper
- 1 tablespoon butter, melted

Instructions

1. Preheat oven to 350 degrees F
2. Over medium-low heat melt butter in a large saucepan. Add onions, garlic and broccoli. Cook slowly, stirring occasionally until the vegetables are soft. Spoon vegetables into crust and sprinkle with cheese.
3. Combine eggs and milk. Season with salt and pepper. Stir in melted butter. Pour egg mixture over vegetables and cheese.
4. Bake in preheated oven for 30 to 50 minutes, or until center has set.

# Strawberry Oatmeal Breakfast Smoothie

Ingredients

- 1 cup soy milk
- 1/2 cup rolled oats
- 1 banana, broken into chunks
- 14 frozen strawberries
- 1/2 teaspoon vanilla extract
- 1 1/2 teaspoons white sugar

Instructions

1. In a blender, combine soy milk, oats, banana and strawberries. Add vanilla and sugar if desired. Blend until smooth. Pour into glasses and serve.

# Baby Spinach Omelet

Ingredients

- 2 eggs
- 1 cup torn baby spinach leaves
- 1 1/2 tablespoons grated Parmesan cheese
- 1/4 teaspoon onion powder
- 1/8 teaspoon ground nutmeg
- salt and pepper to taste

Instructions

1. In a bowl, beat the eggs, and stir in the baby spinach and Parmesan cheese. Season with onion powder, nutmeg, salt, and pepper.
2. In a small skillet coated with cooking spray over medium heat, cook the egg mixture about 3 minutes, until partially set. Flip with a spatula, and continue cooking 2 to 3 minutes. Reduce heat to low, and continue cooking 2 to 3 minutes, or to desired doneness.

# German Potato Pancakes

Ingredients

- 2 eggs
- 2 tablespoons all-purpose flour
- 1/4 teaspoon baking powder
- 1/2 teaspoon salt
- 1/4 teaspoon pepper
- 6 medium potatoes, peeled and shredded
- 1/2 cup finely chopped onion
- 1/4 cup vegetable oil

Instructions

1. In a large bowl, beat together eggs, flour, baking powder, salt, and pepper. Mix in potatoes and onion.
2. Heat oil in a large skillet over medium heat. In batches, drop heaping tablespoonfuls of the potato mixture into the skillet. Press to flatten. Cook about 3 minutes on each side, until browned and crisp. Drain on paper towels.

# Light and Fluffy Spinach Quiche

Ingredients

- 1/2 cup light mayonnaise
- 1/2 cup milk
- 4 eggs, lightly beaten
- 8 ounces shredded reduced-fat Cheddar cheese
- 1 (10 ounce) package frozen chopped spinach, thawed and squeezed dry
- 1/4 cup chopped onion
- 1 (9 inch) unbaked pie shell

Instructions

1. Preheat oven to 400 degrees F. Line a cookie sheet with foil.
2. In a large bowl, whisk together mayonnaise and milk until smooth. Whisk in eggs. Layer spinach, cheese, and onion in pie shell, making several layers of each. Pour in egg mixture. Place quiche on prepared cookie sheet. Cover quiche with foil.
3. Bake in preheated oven for 45 minutes. Remove cover, and bake 10 to 15 minutes, or until top is golden brown and filling is set.

# Make Ahead French Toast

Ingredients

- 5 eggs, lightly beaten
- 1 1/2 cups milk
- 1 cup half-and-half cream
- 1 teaspoon vanilla extract
- 1/2 (1 pound) loaf French bread, cut diagonally in 1 inch slice
- 1/2 cup butter, melted
- 1 cup light brown sugar
- 2 tablespoons maple syrup
- 1 cup chopped pecans

Instructions

1. In a large bowl, whisk together eggs, milk, cream and vanilla. Dip bread slices into egg mixture and place in a lightly greased 9x13 inch baking pan. Refrigerate overnight.
2. The next morning: Preheat oven to 350 degrees F (175 degrees C).
3. In a small bowl, combine butter, sugar, maple syrup and pecans. Spoon mixture over bread.
4. Bake in preheated oven until golden, about 40 minutes. Let stand 5 minutes before serving.

# Purple Monstrosity Fruit Smoothie

Ingredients

- 2 frozen bananas, skins removed and cut in chunks
- 1/2 cup frozen blueberries
- 1 cup orange juice
- 1 tablespoon honey (optional)
- 1 teaspoon vanilla extract (optional)

Instructions

1. Place bananas, blueberries and juice in a blender, puree. Use honey and/or vanilla to taste. Use more or less liquid depending on the thickness you want for your smoothie.

# Baked Omelet Roll

Ingredients

- 6 eggs
- 1 cup milk
- 1/2 cup all-purpose flour
- 1/2 teaspoon salt
- 1/4 teaspoon ground black pepper
- 1 cup shredded Cheddar cheese

Instructions

1. Preheat oven to 450 degrees F (230 degrees C). Lightly grease a 9x13 inch baking pan.
2. In a blender, combine eggs, milk, flour, salt and pepper; cover and process until smooth. Pour into prepared baking pan.
3. Bake in preheated oven until set, about 20 minutes. Sprinkle with cheese.
4. Carefully loosen edges of omelet from pan. Starting from the short edge of the pan, carefully roll up omelet. Place omelet seam side down on a serving plate and cut into 6 equal sized pieces.

# Fluffy Canadian Pancakes

Ingredients

- 1 cup all-purpose flour
- 1 tablespoon baking powder
- 1 cup milk
- 3 egg yolk
- 3 egg whites

Instructions

1. In a medium bowl, combine flour and baking powder. Stir in milk and egg yolk until smooth.
2. In a large glass or metal mixing bowl, beat egg whites until stiff peaks form. Fold 1/3 of the whites into the batter, then quickly fold in remaining whites until no streaks remain.
3. Heat a lightly oiled griddle or frying pan over medium high heat. Pour or scoop the batter onto the griddle, using approximately 1/4 cup for each pancake. Cook until pancakes are golden brown on both sides; serve hot.

# Chapter 2

# 10 Mid-Morning Snacks

# Fluffy Canadian Pancakes

Ingredients

- 1 cup all-purpose flour
- 1 tablespoon baking powder
- 1 cup milk
- 3 egg yolks
- 3 egg whites

Instructions

1. In a medium bowl, combine flour and baking powder. Stir in milk and egg yolk until smooth.
2. In a large glass or metal mixing bowl, beat egg whites until stiff peaks form. Fold 1/3 of the whites into the batter, then quickly fold in remaining whites until no streaks remain.
3. Heat a lightly oiled griddle or frying pan over medium high heat. Pour or scoop the batter onto the griddle, using approximately 1/4 cup for each pancake. Cook until pancakes are golden brown on both sides; serve hot.

# Chocolate Gravy

Ingredients

- 1/2 cup butter
- 4 tablespoons unsweetened cocoa powder
- 1/4 cup all-purpose flour
- 3/4 cup white sugar
- 2 cups milk

Directions

1. Melt butter in a skillet over medium heat. Add cocoa and flour; stir until a thick paste is formed. Stir in sugar and milk. Cook, stirring constantly, until thick.

# Vegetarian Korma

Ingredients

- 1 1/2 tablespoons vegetable oil
- 1 small onion, diced
- 1 teaspoon minced fresh ginger root
- 4 cloves garlic, minced
- 2 potatoes, cubed
- 4 carrots, cubed
- 1 fresh jalapeno pepper, seeded and sliced
- 3 tablespoons ground unsalted cashews
- 1 (4 ounce) can tomato sauce
- 2 teaspoons salt
- 1 1/2 tablespoons curry powder
- 1 cup frozen green peas
- 1/2 green bell pepper, chopped
- 1/2 red bell pepper, chopped
- 1 cup heavy cream
- 1 bunch fresh cilantro for garnish

Instructions

1. Heat the oil in a skillet over medium heat. Stir in the onion, and cook until tender. Mix in ginger and garlic, and continue cooking 1 minute. Mix potatoes, carrots, jalapeno, cashews, and tomato sauce. Season with salt and curry powder. Cook and stir 10 minutes, or until potatoes are tender.
2. Stir peas, green bell pepper, red bell pepper, and cream into the skillet. Reduce heat to low, cover,

and simmer 10 minutes. Garnish with cilantro to serve.

# Home-Fried Potatoes

Ingredients

- 4 red potatoes
- 1 tablespoon olive oil
- 1 onion, chopped
- 1 green bell pepper, seeded and chopped
- 2 tablespoons olive oil
- 1 teaspoon salt
- 3/4 teaspoon paprika
- 1/4 teaspoon ground black pepper
- 1/4 cup chopped fresh parsley

Instructions

1. Bring a large pot of salted water to a boil. Add potatoes and cook until tender but still firm, about 15 minutes. Drain, cool cut into 1/2 inch cubes.
2. In a large skillet, heat 1 tablespoon olive oil over medium high heat. Add onion and green pepper. Cook, stirring often, until soft; about 5 minutes. Transfer to a plate and set aside.
3. Pour remaining 2 tablespoons of oil into the skillet and turn heat to medium-high. Add potato cubes, salt, paprika and black pepper. Cook, stirring occasionally, until potatoes are browned; about 10 minutes. Stir in the onions, green peppers and parsley and cook for another minute. Serve hot.

# Country Style Fried Potatoes

Ingredients

- 1/3 cup shortening
- 6 large potatoes, peeled and cubed
- 1 teaspoon salt
- 1/2 teaspoon ground black pepper
- 1/2 teaspoon garlic powder
- 1/2 teaspoon paprika

Instructions

1. In a large cast iron skillet, heat shortening over medium-high heat. Add potatoes and cook, stirring occasionally, until potatoes are golden brown. Season with salt, pepper, garlic powder and paprika. Serve hot.

# Tomato and Basil Quiche

Ingredients

- 1 tablespoon olive oil
- 1 onion, sliced
- 2 tomatoes, peeled and sliced
- 2 tablespoons all-purpose flour
- 2 teaspoons dried basil
- 3 eggs, beaten
- 1/2 cup milk
- salt and pepper to taste
- 1 (9 inch) unbaked deep dish pie crust
- 1 1/2 cups shredded Colby-Monterey Jack cheese, divided

Directions

1. Preheat oven to 400 degrees F (200 degrees C). Bake pie shell in preheated oven for 8 minutes.
2. Meanwhile, heat olive oil in a large skillet over medium heat. Saute onion until soft; remove from skillet. Sprinkle tomato slices with flour and basil, then saute 1 minute on each side. In a small bowl, whisk together eggs and milk. season with salt and pepper.
3. Spread 1 cup shredded cheese in the bottom of pie crust. Layer onions over cheese, and top with tomatoes. Cover with egg mixture. sprinkle top with remaining 1/2 cup shredded cheese.

4. Bake in preheated oven for 10 minutes. Reduce heat to 350 degrees F (175 degrees C), and bake for 15 to 20 minutes, or until filling is puffed and golden brown. Serve warm.

# Broccoli Quiche with Mashed Potato Crust

Ingredients

- 2 large potatoes, peeled
- 2 cups chopped fresh broccoli
- 1/4 cup milk
- 1/4 teaspoon salt
- 1 tablespoon olive oil
- 1/2 onion, chopped
- 1 cup shredded Cheddar cheese
- 3 eggs
- 1 cup milk
- 1/2 teaspoon salt
- 1/2 teaspoon ground black pepper
- 1/4 teaspoon ground nutmeg

Directions

1. Preheat oven to 350 degrees F
2. Bring a large pot of salted water to a boil. Add potatoes and cook until tender but still firm, about 15 minutes; drain. Meanwhile, place broccoli in a steamer over 1 inch of boiling water, and cover. Cook until tender but still firm, about 2 to 6 minutes. Drain and set aside.
3. Mash the potatoes with milk and salt. Brush a deep 9 inch pie dish with olive oil and press the potatoes in. Brush with remaining olive oil. Bake in

preheated oven for 30 minutes or until lightly browned.

4. Arrange onions, broccoli and cheese in the potato crust. Whisk together the eggs, milk, salt, pepper and nutmeg. Pour over broccoli and cheese.
5. Bake in preheated oven for 30 to 40 minutes, until slightly puffed and cooked throughout. Allow to cool for 10 minutes before serving.

# Apple bites

Ingredients

- 1 apple
- Peanut butter
- Chia seeds

Instructions

1. Slice apple in thin slices
2. Spread peanut butter on the apple slices
3. Sprinkle some chia seeds on the peanut butter
4. Serve with some OJ

# Fruit salad

Ingredients

- 1 sliced apple
- 1 sliced banana
- 1 sliced orange
- 5 sliced strawberries
- Flaxseeds
- Chia seeds

Instructions

1. Mix the apple slices, banana slices, orange slices and strawberry slices in a bowl
2. Sprinkle the top with chia seeds and flaxseeds

# Power Smoothie

Ingredients

- 1 banana
- 1 apple
- Chia seeds
- Flaxseeds
- 1 cup water

Instructions

1. Blend all ingredients
2. serve in a big glass with a straw

# Chapter 3

# 20 Lunch Recipes

# Zucchini Pie

Ingredients

- 3 cups zucchini, diced
- 1 onion, chopped
- 4 eggs, beaten
- 1 cup buttermilk baking mix
- 1/2 cup vegetable oil
- 1/2 cup grated Parmesan cheese
- 1/2 teaspoon dried marjoram
- 1 teaspoon chopped parsley, or to taste
- ground black pepper to taste

Instructions

1. Preheat oven to 350 degrees F (175 degrees C). Grease a 10x6-inch pan or a 12-inch pie plate.
2. In a medium mixing bowl, combine zucchini, onion, eggs, buttermilk baking mix, vegetable oil, Parmesan cheese, marjoram, parsley and pepper; mix well. Spread into the prepared baking dish.
3. Bake for 30 minutes, or until lightly brown.

# Creamy Cheesy Scrambled Eggs with Basil

Ingredients

- 4 eggs
- 3 tablespoons sour cream
- 1/2 cup shredded mozzarella cheese
- salt and pepper to taste
- 2 teaspoons butter
- 1 tablespoon minced fresh basil

Instructions

1. Whisk eggs and sour cream in a bowl until creamy and smooth. Mix in cheese. Season with salt and pepper.
2. Melt butter in a skillet over medium heat. Pour in egg mixture; cook, stirring constantly, until eggs reach the desired consistency. Mix in basil during final minutes of cooking.

# Gnocchi with Mushrooms & Blue Cheese

Ingredients

- 2 x 400g packs fresh gnocchi
- 1 tbsp olive oil
- knob of butter
- 1 large onion roughly chopped
- 500g small Forestière or Portobello mushrooms, sliced
- 2 large garlic cloves, chopped
- 150g pack creamy blue cheese (we used Danish blue)
- small pack parsley (chopped)

Instructions

1. Bring a large pan of water to the boil and cook the gnocchi following pack instructions. When they float to the top of the pan, they are ready. Drain and set aside.
2. Meanwhile, heat the oil and butter in a large lidded frying pan. Add the onion and mushrooms, cook for 1 min over a high heat, then turn down the heat to medium, put the lid on and cook for 5 mins, stirring a few times.
3. Remove the lid and add the garlic, cook for 1-2 mins, then stir the gnocchi into the pan. Scatter over blobs of cheese and the parsley.

# Indian Chickpeas with Poached Eggs

Ingredients

- 1 tbsp rapeseed oil
- 2 garlic cloves, chopped
- 1 yellow pepper, deseeded and diced
- ½ - 1 red chilli, deseeded and chopped
- ½ bunch spring onions (about 5), tops and whites sliced but kept separate
- 1 tsp cumin plus a little extra to serve (optional)
- 1 tsp coriander
- ½ tsp turmeric
- 3 tomatoes cut into wedges
- ⅓ pack coriander, chopped
- 400g can chickpeas in water, drained but liquid reserved
- ½ tsp reduced-salt bouillon powder (we used Marigold)
- 4 large eggs

Instructions

1. Heat the oil in a non-stick sauté pan, add the garlic, pepper, chilli and the whites from the spring onions, and fry for 5 mins over a medium-high heat. Meanwhile, put a large pan of water on to boil.
2. Add the spices, tomatoes, most of the coriander and the chickpeas to the sauté pan and cook for 1-2 mins more. Stir in the bouillon powder and enough

liquid from the chickpeas to moisten everything, and leave to simmer gently.

3. Once the water is at a rolling boil, crack in your eggs and poach for 2 mins, then remove with a slotted spoon. Stir the spring onion tops into the chickpeas, then very lightly crush a few of the chickpeas with a fork or potato masher. Spoon the chickpea mixture onto plates, scatter with the reserved coriander and top with the eggs. Serve with an extra sprinkle of cumin, if you like.

# Hot 'n' spicy roasted red pepper & tomato soup

Ingredients

- 290g roasted red peppers, drained
- 270g cherry tomatoes, halved
- 1 garlic clove, crushed
- 1 vegetable stock cube
- 1 tsp paprika
- 1 tbsp olive oil
- 4 tbsp ground almonds

Instructions

1. Put the roasted red peppers in a blender with the cherry tomatoes, garlic, vegetable stock cube, 100ml water, paprika, olive oil and ground almonds. Blitz until smooth, season well and heat until piping hot before serving.

# Coconut & Squash Dhansak

Ingredients

- 1 tbsp vegetable oil
- 500g butternut squash (about 1 small squash), peeled and chopped into bite-sized chunks (or buy a pack of ready-prepared to save time), see tip, below left
- 100g frozen chopped onions
- 4 heaped tbsp mild curry paste (we used korma)
- 400g can chopped tomatoes
- 400g can light coconut milk
- mini naan bread, to serve
- 400g can lentil (drained)
- 200g bag baby spinach
- 150ml coconut yogurt

Instructions

1. Heat the oil in a large pan. Put the squash in a bowl with a splash of water. Cover with cling film and microwave on High for 10 mins or until tender.
2. Meanwhile, add the onions to the hot oil and cook for a few mins until soft. Add the curry paste, tomatoes and coconut milk, and simmer for 10 mins until thickened to a rich sauce.
3. Warm the naan breads in a low oven or in the toaster.
4. Drain any liquid from the squash, then add to the sauce with the lentils, spinach and some seasoning.

Simmer for a further 2-3 mins to wilt the spinach, then stir in the coconut yogurt.

5. Serve with the warm naan and a dollop of extra yogurt.

# Speedy Mediterranean Gnocchi

Ingredients

- 400g gnocchi
- 200g chargrilled vegetables (from the deli counter - I used chargrilled peppers, aubergines, artichokes and semi-dried tomatoes)
- 2 tbsp red pesto
- a handful of basil leaves
- Parmesan or pecorino (or vegetarian alternative), to serve

Instructions

1. Boil a large pan of salted water. Add the gnocchi, cook for 2 mins or until it rises to the surface, then drain and tip back into the pan with a splash of reserved cooking water.
2. Add the chargrilled veg, chopped into pieces if large, red pesto and basil leaves. Serve with shavings of Parmesan or pecorino (or vegetarian alternative).

# Sweetcorn & Courgetti Fritters

Ingredients

- 200g can sweetcorn (drained)
- 2 spring onions, finely chopped
- 50g courgetti (grated)
- 1 tsp smoked paprika
- 50g self-raising flour
- 5 eggs, 1 beaten, 4 for poaching
- 40ml milk
- 4 tbsp sweet chilli sauce
- juice 1 lime
- 1 tbsp vegetable oil
- mixed leaves, to serve

Instructions

1. Mix the sweetcorn, spring onions, courgetti, paprika, flour, beaten egg, milk and some seasoning in a large bowl and set aside.
2. Put a large pan of water on to boil. In a bowl, mix the chilli sauce with the lime juice and set aside.
3. Heat the oil in a large, non-stick pan and spoon in four burger-sized mounds of the fritter mixture, spaced apart (you may need to do this in two batches). When brown on the underside, turn over and cook for 3 mins more until golden.
4. Meanwhile, poach the eggs in the simmering water for 2-3 mins until cooked and the yolks are runny. Remove with a slotted spoon. Serve the fritters

topped with a poached egg, mixed leaves and a drizzle of the chilli dressing.

# Boiled Egg, Avocado & Quick Pickled Radish Tartine

## Ingredients

- 100g mixed radishes cut into different shapes
- 1 tbsp white wine vinegar
- pinch caster sugar
- 1 large avocado
- juice ½ lime
- pinch chilli flakes
- 4 slices of your favourite bread (we used sourdough)
- 2 eggs, soft boiled for 6 mins, then rinsed under cold water, peeled and halved)

## Instructions

2. Toss the radishes in a bowl with the vinegar, sugar and a pinch of salt. In a separate bowl, mash the avocado with the lime juice, chilli flakes and some seasoning. Toast the bread, then top each slice with a little avocado, half an egg, some pickled radishes and a few more chilli flakes, if you like.

# Grilled Peach Panzanella

Ingredients

- 3 banana shallots, finely sliced into rings
- 2 tbsp cider vinegar
- pinch of golden caster sugar
- 3 firm peaches, halved, flat peaches are nice, if you can get them
- 3 ½ tbsp extra virgin olive oil
- pinch of red chilli flakes
- pinch of fennel seeds
- juice ½ lemon
- 1 tbsp capers (rinsed)
- 2 slices day-old sourdough, torn into chunks
- handful wild rocket
- small pack basil, leaves picked
- fennel fronds, from the crispy pork belly recipe (optional)

Instructions

1. Quick-pickle the shallots in a bowl with the cider vinegar and sugar. Destone and slice the peaches.
2. Put the peaches in a bowl and toss with 1/2 tbsp olive oil, the chilli flakes, fennel seeds and some seasoning. Heat a griddle pan over a high heat and sear the peaches for 2 mins each side until they have char lines on them. Remove from the heat and allow to cool.

3.  Pour the vinegar from the shallots into a bowl and whisk together with the remaining olive oil and some seasoning to make a dressing.
4.  Put the peaches in a salad bowl or sharing platter with the lemon juice, shallots, capers and bread, season well and pour over the dressing. Add the rocket, basil and fennel fronds (if using), and toss thoroughly with your hands to combine.

# Pineapple and Avocado Salad

Ingredients

- ¼ cup red onion (sliced)
- Ice water
- 2 ripe avocados (sliced)
- 1 medium pineapple (sliced)
- 3 tablespoons olive oil
- 1 tablespoon lime juice
- ½ teaspoon kosher salt
- ½ teaspoon ground pepper
- ½ flaxseeds

Instructions

1. Pour ice water and onion in a large bowl and let soak for 10-15 minutes
2. Drain the onion slices
3. Mix avocado, pineapple, onion, oil and lime juice in a bowl
4. Add salt to the mixture
5. Sprinkle the top with flaxseeds

# Veggie Chinese Pancakes

## Ingredients

- 200g mushroom, sliced (we used chestnut)
- 2 tbsp soy sauce
- ½ tsp five spice powder
- 1 tbsp rice wine, preferably Shaohsing
- ½ tbsp sesame oil
- 1 tsp sugar
- 6 Chinese pancakes
- 2 spring onions (sliced)
- 5cm length cucumber, deseeded and sliced into matchsticks
- ½ Little Gem lettuce, shredded
- 4 tbsp hoisin sauce

## Instructions

1. Heat a small frying pan. Add the mushrooms, soy, five-spice, rice wine, sesame oil and sugar. Stir until the mushrooms are cooked and the sauce is thick, bubbling and clinging to the mushrooms. Warm the pancakes – steam them or heat them in the microwave.
2. Serve the mushrooms, spring onions, cucumber, lettuce and hoisin sauce in separate dishes, with the pancakes alongside.
3. To assemble, spread a pancake, with a little hoisin sauce. Add some mushrooms, onions, cucumber and lettuce. Fold the pancake and enjoy.

# Black Bean Soup

Ingredients

- 1 tablespoon canola oil
- 1 small onion (chopped)
- 1 tablespoon chili powder
- 1 teaspoon cumin
- 2 15-ounce cans black beans
- 3 cups water
- ¼ teaspoon salt
- 1 tablespoon lime juice
- 2 tablespoons cilantro (chopped)
- ½ chia seeds

Instructions

1. Mix oil, onion, chili powder, cumin in a saucepan over medium heat
2. Wait 2 minutes and then add beans, water and salt
3. Bring to boil and cook for 10 minutes over low-medium heat
4. Once cooked, transfer the soup to a blender and blend until smooth
5. Serve on a plate with cilantro and sprinkle soup with chia seeds

# Spicy Courgetti Pitta Pockets

Ingredients

- 1 courgetti, trimmed and thinly sliced lengthways
- 2 tsp harissa paste
- 2 tsp olive oil
- small handful broad beans
- 2 tbsp houmous
- 1 spring onion (sliced)
- 1 tsp tahini paste
- small garlic clove, crushed
- squeeze lemon juice
- 1 tbsp Greek-style yogurt
- yogurtYogurt yog-ert
- Yogurt is made by adding a number of types of harmless bacteria to milk, causing it to ferment....
- 1 large wholemeal pitta bread

Instructions

1. Toss the courgette slices in the harissa and olive oil, and season. Cook on a hot griddle pan for 2 mins each side or until tender. Transfer to a plate and set aside.
2. Cook the broad beans in boiling water for 2 mins, drain under cold running water, then slip them out of their outer skins. Discard the skins. Put the broad beans, houmous and spring onion in a small bowl and mix to combine.

3.  In another bowl, mix the tahini, garlic, lemon juice and yogurt. Toast the pitta and split it to create 2 pockets. Spoon the houmous mix inside each pocket, followed by the spicy courgette slices and a drizzle of the yogurt mixture.

# Asparagus & Courgetti Salad with Feta & Sesame Seeds

## Ingredients

- 1 tsp sesame seed
- 140g asparagus
- 50g pea
- 200g courgetti
- 1 tsp sesame or olive oil
- small handful rocket leaves
- 20g feta cheese
- grated zest ½ lemon

## Instructions

1. Heat a small frying pan and add the sesame seeds. Cook, shaking the pan and making sure the seeds don't burn. When they are fragrant and have turned a light teak color, tip them onto a saucer.
2. Steam the asparagus for 3-4 mins until almost done. Drop into a bowl of iced water to cool, then drain and wrap in a tea towel to dry really well. Cook the peas for 3 mins in the boiling water used to steam the asparagus, then drain and cool under a cold tap. Slice the courgetti on the diagonal, about 0.5cm thick.
3. Heat a griddle pan until very hot. Brush the asparagus and courgetti slices with the oil, and cook in batches until nicely striped with dark brown. Cut the asparagus into 5cm lengths.

# Carrot & ginger immune-boosting soup

Ingredients

- 3 large carrots
- 1 tbsp grated ginger
- 1 tsp turmeric
- a pinch of cayenne pepper, plus extra to serve
- 20g wholemeal bread
- 1 tbsp soured cream, plus extra to serve
- 200ml vegetable stock

Instructions

1. Peel and chop the carrots and put in a blender with the ginger, turmeric, cayenne pepper, wholemeal bread, soured cream and vegetable stock. Blitz until smooth. Heat until piping hot. Swirl through some extra soured cream, or a sprinkling of cayenne, if you like.

4. Mix the asparagus, courgettes, peas, rocket, feta and lemon zest. Grind over some black pepper and sprinkle with the sesame seeds before serving.

# Artichoke & Roasted Red Repper Souffle Omelette

Ingredients

- 5 eggs
- , separated
- 2 whole eggs
- ½ can artichoke hearts, drained, quartered if whole
- 1 whole roasted pepper
- from a jar or can drained, patted dry and roughly chopped
- 50g vegetarian Parmesan-style cheese
- 10 large basil leaves, shredded
- 1 tbsp butter
- 1 tbsp extra virgin rapeseed or olive oil

Instructions

1. In a large bowl, lightly beat together the 5 egg yolks and 2 whole eggs. In a separate bowl, use an electric whisk to beat the egg whites until stiff. Add whites to the yolks and fold together carefully, keeping it light and fluffy. Fold in the artichokes, pepper, half the cheese, the basil, salt and pepper.
2. Heat grill to high. Heat a medium non-stick frying pan over a medium heat. Add the butter and oil. When the butter has melted, add the omelette mixture and spread evenly.
3. Cook until golden underneath, about 5 mins. Scatter over remaining cheese, then place the pan under

the grill and cook for a further 2 mins. Slide the omelette onto a board or serving plate.

4. Cut into wedges and serve.

# Gujarati Cabbage with Coconut & Potato

## Ingredients

- 500g Charlotte or other new potato
- 2 tbsp sunflower oil
- 1 pinch asafoetida
- 1 tsp black mustard seeds
- 1 tsp cumin seeds
- 2 dried red chillies
- 1 fresh red or green chilli, deseeded and thinly sliced
- 1 pointed (sweetheart) cabbage (shredded)
- juice ½ lemon
- 2 tbsp desiccated or shaved fresh coconut (toasted)
- bunch of coriander, roughly chopped

## Instructions

1. Cook potatoes in a pan of salted boiling water for 10 mins until tender. Drain well and return to pan. Lightly crush with the back of a fork, just to break, not to mash.
2. Heat the oil in a large frying pan and then add the asafoetida, spices and dried chillies. Cook for a few mins until the spices pop and the chillies darken.
3. Add the fresh chilli, cabbage and some salt and stir-fry for 3-4 mins. Add the warm potatoes to the pan and cook for 2-3 mins more until the cabbage is

tender, but still has some bite. Stir in the lemon juice, coconut and coriander, and serve.

# Bulghar & Broad Bean Salad with Zesty Dressing

Ingredients

- 50g bulghar wheat
- 85g frozen broad bean, defrosted and podded, if you like
- 6 sugar snap pea, halved lengthways
- 4 radish (sliced)
- ½ small red onion, thinly sliced
- small handful mint leaves

For the dressing

- zest and juice 1 lime
- ½ small red chilli, deseeded and chopped
- 1 tbsp extra-virgin olive oil
- 1 tsp white wine vinegar
- 1 tsp clear honey

Instructions

1. Cook the bulghar wheat following pack instructions, adding the broad beans for the final 2 mins. Cool under cold running water, drain well, then toss with the sugar snap peas, radishes and red onion.
2. Whisk together the dressing ingredients with some seasoning and toss through the salad. Scatter with the mint leaves.

# Tex-Mex burrito

Ingredients

- 2 tomatoes (chopped)
- 3 spring onions (chopped)
- 1 red chilli, sliced (deseeded if you like it milder)
- 4 eggs
- 100ml milk
- 1 tsp olive oil
- 100g cheddar (grated)
- 2 large wraps
- soured cream and guacamole to serve, (optional)

Instructions

1. In a small bowl, mix the tomatoes, half the spring onions and half the red chilli with some seasoning and set aside. Beat the eggs and milk with a fork with some seasoning.
2. Heat the oil in a large non-stick pan and fry the remaining spring onion and chilli for 1 min, then pour in the egg mix. Gently scramble the eggs by dragging the egg mixture as it sets into the middle of the pan
3. Cook to your liking, then take off the heat and throw on the cheese. Stir through, then divide between the wraps
4. Tuck up the top and bottom of each wrap and roll up, then slice in half and serve with the homemade tomato salsa, soured cream and guacamole, if you like.

# Chapter 4

# 20 Dinner Recipes

# Chili with Pesto

Ingredients

- 1 tablespoon olive oil
- 1 small yellow onion (chopped)
- 2 carrots (diced)
- 11 4.5-ounce can tomatoes (diced)
- Kosher salt
- Black pepper
- 1 can chickpeas
- 1 can cannellini beans
- 1 can of lentils
- 1 can kidney beans
- 1 clove garlic (chopped)
- 3 tablespoons pine nuts (chopped)
- 1cup parsley (chopped)
- 2 cup water

Instructions

1. In a saucepan min oil, onion and carrots over medium heat and sauté for 5 minutes
2. Pour tomatoes, water, salt and pepper in the saucepan and bring to boil
3. Add chickpeas, cannellini beans, kidney beans and lentils and cook for about 5 minutes
4. Mix garlic, nuts, parsley, oil, salt and pepper in a small bowl and mix until all ingredients are well mixed (pesto)

5. Pour chili in large bowl and add pesto on the top before serving

# Creamy Vegan Garlic Pasta

Ingredients

- 10 ounces whole wheat pasta
- Olive oil
- 2 medium shallots (diced)
- 8 large cloves garlic (minced)
- Salt
- Black pepper
- 2 1/2 cups vegan milk (almond suggested)

Instructions

1. Cook pasta according to package instructions
2. Mix vegan milk, 1 tablespoon olive oil, garlic and shallot in a saucepan and cook over medium heat for 3 minutes (sauce)
3. Drain pasta when ready and transfer into a bowl
4. Pour sauce on top and mix well
5. Sprinkle with black pepper before serving

# Cauliflower Fettuccine

Ingredients

- 4 heaping cups steamed cauliflower florets
- 1/2 tablespoon olive oil
- 1 tablespoon garlic clove (minced)
- 1/2 cup vegan milk (almond suggested)
- 1/4 cup nutritional yeast
- 1 tablespoon lemon juice
- ½ teaspoon onion powder
- ¾ teaspoon salt
- ¼ teaspoon pepper
- Fettuccine pasta
- Fresh parsley

Instructions

1. Add oil and garlic in a saucepan over medium heat and sauté until garlic is fragrant
2. In a blender mix cauliflower, sautéed garlic, vegan milk, nutritional yeast, lemon juice, onion powder, salt and pepper and blend until sauce is smooth (sauce)
3. Cook pasta according to package instructions
4. Drain pasta when ready and transfer into a bowl
5. Pour sauce on top and mix well
6. Sprinkle parsley and black pepper on top before serving

# Curried Eggplant

Ingredients

- 1 cup basmati rice (steamed)
- ½ teaspoon salt
- ½ teaspoon black pepper
- 1 tablespoon olive oil
- 1 onion (chopped)
- 1 medium size eggplant (chopped)
- 1 ½teaspoons curry powder
- 11 5.5-ounce can chickpeas
- ½ cup basil
- 2 cups water

Instructions

1. Mix oil and garlic in a saucepan over medium heat and sauté until garlic is fragrant
2. Add eggplant, curry powder, salt and black pepper in the saucepan and cook for a couple of minutes
3. Add water and cook for 10-15 minutes
4. Add chickpeas and cook for another 5 minutes
5. Spread the rice over the plate and pour the vegetables on the to
6. Sprinkle with basil before serving

# Black Beans and Rice

Ingredients

- Kosher salt
- 2 1/2tablespoons olive oil
- 2 cups long-grain rice (cooked)
- 1 medium onion (chopped)
- 1 large red pepper (chopped)
- 2 medium cloves garlic (chopped)
- 2 15-ounce cans black beans
- 1 cup vegetable or chicken broth
- 2 tablespoons red wine vinegar
- ½ teaspoon ground black pepper
- ¼ teaspoon ground cumin

Instructions

1. In sauce pan mix oil, onion, red pepper and garlic and sauté for about 5 minutes
2. Add beans, broth, vinegar, black pepper, cumin and salt and bring to boil
3. Cook for about 10 minutes
4. Spread the rice over the plate and pour the beans over the top
5. Serve with favorite vegetables

# Winter Lentil Soup

## Ingredients

- 1 tablespoon olive oil
- 4 broccoli (chopped)
- 1 28-ounce can whole tomatoes (chopped)
- 2 sweet potatoes (sliced)
- 1 bunch kale (chopped)
- ½ cup lentils
- 1 tablespoon thyme
- Kosher salt
- Black pepper
- 6 cups water
- ½ tablespoon chia seeds

## Instructions

1. Mix oil and broccoli in saucepan and cook for a few minutes over medium heat
2. Add tomatoes and cook for another 5 minutes
3. Add water and bring to boil
4. Add the sweet potatoes, kale, lentils, thyme, 1 ½ teaspoons salt, and ¼ teaspoon pepper
5. Cook for approximately 30 minutes
6. Pour lentils into a bowl and sprinkle with chia seeds before serving

# Spicy Coconut Noodles

Ingredients

- 8 ounces rice noodles
- 11 3.5-ounce coconut milk
- 1 teaspoon chili powder
- 1 teaspoon kosher salt
- 1 tablespoon chili paste
- Basil leaves
- Chili paste

Instructions

1. Cook noodles according to the package directions
2. Mix coconut milk, chili powder, salt, and chili paste in a saucepan and bring to boil
3. Drain noodles and pour into the saucepan
4. Cook for a couple of minutes. Make sure all ingredients are well mixed
5. Top with basil leaves before serving

# Stir-Fried Rice Noodles with Tofu and Vegetables

## Ingredients

- 18-ounce package rice noodles
- ¼ cup brown sugar
- ¼ cup soy sauce
- 2 tablespoons lime juice
- 11 4-ounce package firm tofu (sliced into small cubes)
- 1 tablespoon canola oil
- 2 carrots (thinly sliced)
- 1 red bell pepper (thinly sliced)
- 1 tablespoon ginger
- 2 cups bean sprouts
- 4 scallions (thinly sliced)
- ¼ cup roasted peanuts (chopped)

## Instructions

1. Cook noodles according to package directions
2. Mix together sugar, soy sauce and lime juice in a small bowl
3. Mix oil, tofu, carrots, bell pepper and ginger in a large pan and sauté for a couple of minutes
4. Add the soy sauce mix and the noodles into the pan and cook for 1-2 minutes over low-medium heat

5. Transfer the noodles into a plate and sprinkle scallion and peanuts over the top before serving

# Vegan Fajitas

Ingredients

- 1 poblano pepper (sliced)
- 2 bell peppers (sliced)
- 1 jalapeño, seeds removed (sliced)
- 1 white onion (chopped)
- 2 large portobello mushrooms (sliced)
- 2 ripe avocados
- 1/2 lime juice
- ½ teaspoon sea salt
- ½ teaspoon cumin
- ½ teaspoon garlic powder
- 6 small flour tortillas
- Hot sauce
- Olive oil

Instructions

1. Mix oil, onion and pepper in a skillet over medium-high heat and sauté until fragrant
2. While cooking add salt, cumin and garlic powder
3. Mix oil and mushrooms in a pan and sauté
4. Mix avocados, lime juice and salt into a bowl and mix until smooth
5. Warm tortillas before serving

# Peanut Noodles

Ingredients

- ¼ cup peanut butter
- 1.5 tablespoons sesame oil
- 1 teaspoon soy sauce
- 1.5 teaspoons lime
- ½ teaspoon grated ginger
- 1 teaspoon sriracha
- ¼ cup water
- 8 oz. noodles
- Eggplant
- Red peppers
- Scallions (chopped)
- Sesame seeds
- Crushed peanuts
- Chia seeds

Instructions

1. Mix peanut butter, soy sauce, sesame oil, lime juice, ginger, siracha, and water in a small bowl
2. Cook noodles according to package directions
3. Drain noodles and set aside
4. Mix oil, eggplant, red pepper and scallion in a skillet over medium heat
5. Add noodles and cook for a couple of minutes
6. Sprinkle with sesame seeds, chia seeds and peanuts before serving

# Chickpea Veggie Burger

Ingredients

- 1 can chickpeas (mashed)
- ½ red onion (diced)
- 1 small zucchini (sliced)
- 3 tablespoon cilantro (chopped)
- 3 tablespoon vinegar
- 1 tablespoon sriracha sauce
- 2 tablespoon peanut butter
- 1 tsp cumin
- 1 tsp garlic powder
- 2 tsp black pepper
- ½ tsp sea salt
- 2 tbsp. olive oil

Instructions

1. Mash chickpeas in a bowl.
2. Add all ingredients into the bowl and mix until all ingredients are well mixed
3. Form small patties
4. Cook burgers in a skillet with olive oil for a couple of minutes on each side
5. Serve with favorite sides

# Sweet and Spicy Asian Tofu

Ingredients

- 7 ounces extra firm tofu (sliced into small cubes)
- 1 tablespoon olive oil
- Cooking spray
- 1 clove garlic (minced)
- 3 cups assorted stir-fry vegetables
- 3 tablespoons sweet chili sauce
- 2 tablespoons Sriracha hot sauce
- 2 teaspoons soy sauce
- ⅔ cup brown rice (cooked)
- 1 tablespoon chia seeds

Instructions

1. Mix oil and tofu in a pan and sauté until golden color is reached
2. Mix oil, garlic and vegetables in a different pan and sauté until fragrant
3. Add tofu, chili sauce and hot sauce into the second pan and cook for a few minutes
4. Spread brown rice on a plate and pour tofu and vegetables on top of it
5. Sprinkle chia seeds over the top before serving

# Quinoa Edamame Salad

Ingredients

- 2 cups shelled edamame (steamed)
- 1 cup quinoa (cooked)
- 1 green onion (sliced)
- ½ red bell pepper (diced)
- 2 Tablespoon cilantro (chopped)
- 1½ Tablespoon olive oil
- 1 Tablespoon lemon juice
- ¼ tsp salt
- ¼ tsp chili powder
- ¼ tsp dried thyme
- ⅛ tsp ground black pepper
- Pinch of cayenne

Instructions

1. Mix edamame, quinoa, green onion, red pepper and cilantro in a large bowl
2. Mix oil, lemon juice, salt, chili powder, black pepper, thyme and cayenne in a small bowl (dressing)
3. Pour the dressing over quinoa before serving

# White Bean Vegetables Soup

Ingredients

- 1 Tablespoon olive oil
- 1 medium onion (diced)
- 2 medium carrots (diced)
- 2 celery ribs (diced)
- 1 large leek (sliced)
- 2 cloves garlic (chopped)
- 3 Tablespoons tomato paste
- 1½ cups cooked white beans
- 1 28 ounce can diced tomatoes
- 6-8 cups vegetable broth
- 2 sprigs thyme
- 4-5 kale leaves (chopped)
- Salt
- Ground black pepper
- Chia seeds

Instructions

1. Mix oil, onion, carrots, celery, leeks, garlic, tomato paste, beans, diced tomatoes, broth, thyme, salt and pepper in a soup pot and cook for about 15 minutes
2. Add kale and cook for another 10 minutes
3. Serve into a bowl and sprinkle with chia seeds

# Vegan mac and cheese

Ingredients

- 14 ounces cooked pasta
- 3 tablespoons vegan butter
- 1/4 cup whole wheat flour
- 2 cups vegan milk (almond suggested)
- 1-1/2 cup vegan cheese
- 1 cup vegan cheddar cheese
- Salt
- Pepper

Instructions

1. Preheat oven to 350 F
2. Grease a backing dish and set aside
3. Mix flour, salt and margarine in a large saucepan over medium heat
4. Slowly add milk and reduce heat
5. Add pasta and mix
6. Pour pasta into the backing dish and cook for 15-20 minutes
7. Serve with vegan cheese

# Vegan Vodka Pasta

Ingredients

- 2 tablespoons olive oil
- 1/4 cup white onion (diced)
- 2 garlic cloves (minced)
- 2 tablespoons tomato paste
- 1 pint cherry tomatoes (diced)
- 1/4 teaspoon red pepper flakes
- 1/4 teaspoon ground black pepper
- 1/4 teaspoon salt
- 1/3 cup vodka
- 1/2 cup vegan milk
- 1/3 cup vegan cheese
- 2 tablespoons vegan butter
- 8 ounces penne pasta (cooked)

Instructions

1. Mix oil, onion, garlic and tomato paste in a large pot over medium heat and sauté until fragrant
2. Add salt, pepper, tomatoes and red pepper and cook for a couple of minutes
3. Add vodka and cook for another 5 minutes
4. Pour in milk, cheese and butter and cook for a few more minutes
5. Add pasta and stir to combine
6. Sprinkle with vegan cheese before serving

# Quesadilla

Ingredients

- 1/2 avocado
- 2 tortillas 1 tomato (chopped)
- 2 tbsp. chives
- 1 tsp nutritional yeast

Instructions

1. Mash avocado and spread it on a tortilla
2. Sprinkle a bit of yeast and chives
3. Add tomatoes and place the second tortilla on top
4. Place your quesadilla inside a pan over medium heat and cook each side until golden

# Broccoli Walnut Pesto Pasta

Ingredients

- 1 large head of broccoli, florets only (steamed)
- Pinch of salt
- 16 oz. of pasta
- 1/3 cup of walnuts (chopped)
- 2 garlic cloves (whole)
- 1 Tbsp. fresh basil
- 1 Tbsp. lemon juice
- 1 Tbsp. olive oil
- 1 tsp. apple cider vinegar

Instructions

1. Cook pasta according to package directions
2. Mix walnuts, garlic, basil, lemon juice, olive oil and vinegar in a food processor and process until smooth
3. Add broccoli florets to the processor and process until smooth
4. Drain pasta and, in a large bowl, combine pasta and pesto sauce
5. Sprinkle with crushed walnuts on top before serving

# Vegan Bolognese Pasta

Ingredients

- 1 ½ cups lentils (cooked)
- 3 cups water
- 1 Tbs. vegetable oil
- 1 large yellow onion (diced)
- 2 bell peppers (diced)
- 4 cloves garlic (minced)
- 3 Tbs. tomato paste
- 28 oz. diced tomatoes
- 1 tsp. ground fennel
- 1 tsp. dried oregano
- 1 tsp. paprika
- Pinch of red pepper flakes
- Kosher salt
- Black pepper
- 1-lb. pasta
- Fresh basil leaves

Instructions

1. Mash lentils in a bowl
2. Cook pasta according to package instructions
3. Heat oil in a large saucepan over medium heat and add mashed lentils. Cook for 5 minutes
4. Add onions, peppers, garlic and tomato paste in the saucepan and cook for 5 more minutes

5. Add in the diced tomatoes, fennel, oregano, paprika, and red pepper flakes and cook over low heat for 5-10 minutes. Add water in needed
6. Drain pasta and, in a large bowl, mix pasta and sauce until well mixed
7. Sprinkle with basil before serving

# Black Beans and Rice

Ingredients

- Kosher salt 2 ½ tbsp.
- Olive oil
- 2 cups rice (cooked)
- 1 medium onion (chopped)
- 1 large red pepper (chopped)
- 2 medium cloves garlic (chopped)
- 2 15 oz. cans black beans
- 1 cup vegetable
- 2 tbsp. red wine
- 2 bay leaves
- ½ tsp freshly ground black pepper
- ¼ tsp ground cumin
- ½ cup scallions (sliced)

Instructions

1. Mix oil, onions, garlic and red pepper in saucepan and sauté for 5 minutes over medium heat
2. Add broth, vinegar, bay leaves, beans, black pepper, salt and cumin Cover with a lid and bring to boil
3. Lower heat and simmer for 10 minutes before removing bay leaves
4. Take rice out in a plate or bowl and pour beans over the rice
5. Sprinkle with salt and pepper if needed before serving

# Chapter 5

# 20 Dessert Recipes

# Power Cookies

Ingredients

- 4 cups rolled oats
- 1 can cannellini beans
- ½ cup white sugar
- ½ cup brown sugar
- 1 teaspoon vanilla extract
- 1 teaspoon baking powder
- 1 teaspoon baking soda
- 1 teaspoon ground cinnamon
- ½ cup pitted dates (chopped)
- 1/2 cup flaked coconut
- 1/2 cup raisins
- 1/2 cup walnuts (chopped)

Instructions

1. Preheat oven to 330 F
2. Pour oats into a blender and blend until it turn onto flour
3. Mash beans in a bowl
4. Add sugar and vanilla and mix
5. Combine the ground oats, baking powder, baking soda and cinnamon, blend into the bean mixture
6. Stir in the dates, coconut, raisins and walnuts
7. Make cookies with your hands and bake for 15 minutes
8. Let cool before serving

# Vegan Chocolate Truffles

Ingredients

- 2 cups soft dates (pitted)
- 1 and 1/2 tablespoons cocoa powder
- 3 tablespoons orange juice

Instructions

1. Mix dates, cocoa powder and oj in a blender and blend until smooth
2. Make small balls and mix it with cocoa powder
3. Place truffles on a plate before serving

# Flowerless Brownies

Ingredients

- 3 medium ripe bananas
- 1/2 cup smooth peanut butter
- 2 T - 1/4 cup cocoa powder

Instructions

1. Preheat oven to 350 F
2. Grease a pan and set aside
3. Melt butter in the microwave
4. Mix bananas, butter and cocoa butter in a bowl and mix
5. Pour brownie mixture into the pan and cook for 20 minutes
6. Slice before serving

# Vegan Fudge

Ingredients

- 1 heaped cup mini chocolate chips
- 1/2 cup solidified coconut butter
- 1 teaspoon vanilla

Instructions

1. Pour chocolate chips into a bowl and melt in the microwave
2. Pour butter into the melted chocolate and mix
3. Stir in vanilla and keep mixing
4. Pour in a clear plastic wrap and refrigerate for 1 hour
5. Slice before serving

# Chocolate Avocado Pudding

Ingredients

- 2 large avocados
- 1/2 cup cocoa
- 1/2 cup maple syrup
- ¼ cup almond milk

Instructions

1. Mix all ingredients into blender and blend until smooth
2. Pour into small cups before serving

# Cacao Bites

Ingredients

- 1 cup walnuts
- 1 cup dates
- 2 tbsp. raw cacao

Instructions

1. Crush walnuts using a blender
2. Add dates and cacao into the blender and mix
3. Make small balls with your hands before serving

# Apple Strudel

Ingredients

- 1 package vegan puff pastry dough
- 2 apples
- ¾ teaspoon cinnamon
- Powdered sugar

Instructions

1. Preheat oven to 350 F
2. Slice apples into thin slices
3. Mix apple slices and cinnamon in a bowl
4. Put apple slices on the pastry dough and fold it in
5. Cook for about 15 minutes
6. Sprinkle with powdered sugar before serving

# Oatmeal Cookies

Ingredients

- 2 large ripe bananas (peeled)
- 1 cup rolled oats

Instructions

1. Preheat oven to 350 F
2. Grease a baking sheet with cooking spray
3. Mash bananas in a bowl and add oats
4. Make cookies with your hands
5. Put cookies onto baking sheet
6. Bake for 15 minutes
7. Let cool before serving

# Almond Butter Cups

Ingredients

- 200 grams dark chocolate squares
- 3/4 cups almond butter
- 4 tablespoons of coconut oil (divided)

Instructions

1. Melt chocolate in the microwave
2. Pour water onto a pot and bring to boil
3. Pour in chocolate and 2 tbsp. of coconut oil and melt completely
4. Mix butter and 2 tbsp. coconut oil in a bowl
5. Line a flat dish with muffin or cupcake liners
6. With a spoon, scoop in a little melted chocolate to cover the bottom of each liner
7. Place in the freezer for about 2 minute to slightly set
8. Add a small scoop of butter and coconut butter mix in the center and gently flatten with the back of a spoon
9. Scoop more melted chocolate to cover the top, about 1-2 tablespoons
10. Freeze for about 15-30 minutes before serving

# Mulberry Cookies

Ingredients

- ½ cup dried white mulberries
- 5 large medjool dates
- 2½ - 3 tbsp coconut (shredded)

Instructions

1. Blend all ingredients in a blender until you get a smooth dough
2. Scoop out about 1 tablespoon of mixture, roll into a ball then flatten into a cookie shape
3. Let rest for 10 minutes before serving

# Almond Butter Fudge

## Ingredients

- 1/2 cup coconut butter
- 1/3 cup creamy almond butter
- 2 tablespoons pure maple syrup

## Instructions

1. Add all three ingredients to a double boiler. Heat for 4-5 minutes, stirring constantly, or until completely melted together
2. Grease a small 4x6 pan or container with coconut oil and pour the mixture into it. Drop the container on the counter a few times to smooth out the top of the fudge
3. Refrigerate for 2 hours or until set. Turn container over and tap to release the fudge. Slice and enjoy
4. Store in refrigerator

# Banana Peanut Butter Ice Cream

Ingredients

- 4 large very ripe bananas
- 2 tablespoons peanut butter

Instructions

1. Slice bananas and arrage it on a plate
2. Freeze for about 2 hours
3. Blend frozen bananas in a food processor until smooth
4. Add peanut butter and mix
5. Serve right away or freeze

# Peanut Butter Cookies

Ingredients

- 1 cup creamy peanut butter
- 1 cup sugar
- 3 tablespoons chia seeds mixed with 6 tablespoons water and stirred well (eggs)

Instructions

1. Preheat oven to 350 F
2. Mix all ingredients in a bowl with your hands until smooth
3. Make cookies and spread it on cooking sheets
4. Bake for 10 minutes
5. Let cool before serving

# Vegan Nutella Cookies

Ingredients

- 1 1/2 cups oats
- 2 very ripe bananas
- 6 tbsp dairy-free nutella

Instructions

1. Preheat the oven to 350 degrees
2. Mash the bananas in a bowl
3. Add the oats and nutella and mix until smooth
4. Make cookies with your hands and scoop it onto the baking sheet
5. Bake for 15 minutes
6. Let cool before serving

# Coffee Ice Cream

Ingredients

- 1 cup vegan milk
- 1 tsp instant coffee
- Sweetener

Instructions

1. Mix coffee, sweetener and milk in a bowl
2. Blend ice cream with ice cubes in a food processor
3. Serve into small cups

# Vegan Cheesecake

Ingredients

- Cooking spray
- 18 vegan biscuits
- 3 tablespoons sugar
- 3 tablespoons vegan margarine
- 1 1/2 pounds extra firm silken tofu
- 1 pound vegan cream cheese
- 1 1/2 cups sugar
- 1 tablespoon cornflour
- 1 tablespoon pure vanilla extract
- 1 tablespoon freshly squeezed lemon juice
- 1 tablespoon freshly squeezed orange juice
- 2 cups fresh raspberries

Instructions

1. Preheat oven to 350 F
2. Spray a springform pan with cooking spray
3. Mix biscuits and sugar in a food processor until crumbs form
4. Add margarine and 2 tbsp. water in a bowl and melt in the microwave
5. Pour in crumbs into bowland mix
6. Pour mixture into the prepared pan
7. Bake for about 15 minutes
8. Let cool for 20 minutes
9. Blend tofu in a food processor for about 2 minutes

10. Add cheese, sugar, flour, cornflour, vanilla, lemon juice and blende for 2 minutes
11. Pour into crust
12. Bake cheesecake for about 1 hour
13. Let cool for 1 hour before serving

# Carrot Cake

Ingredients

- 1 cup whole wheat flour
- 1 tsp cinnamon
- 1/2 tsp baking powder
- 1 tsp baking soda
- 3/4 cup brown sugar
- 1/2 cup chopped walnuts
- 1/2 tsp allspice
- 1/4 tsp salt
- 1 tsp vanilla extract
- 3 tbsp. safflower oil
- 1/4 cup almond milk, unsweetened
- 1 cup shredded carrots
- 1 cup of tofu cream cheese
- 1/2 tsp vanilla extract
- 2 tsp agave syrup

Instructions

1. Preheat oven to 350 F.
2. Mix whole wheat flour, brown sugar, cinnamon, baking soda, baking powder, allspice, walnuts and salt into a large mixing bowl and mix well
3. Pour the almond milk into another separate mixing bowl and add vanilla extract, safflower oil, grated carrots and mix well
4. Add almond milk mixture to the other mixing bowl

5. Mix well and pour into a round cake pan
6. Bake for 35 minutes
7. Mix tofu cream, vanilla extract and agave syrup in bowl (frosting)
8. Apply frosting to cake once cake cooled down

# Coconut Truffles

Ingredients

- 3/4 cup flour
- 3 cups unsweetened coconut (shredded)
- 1 cup sugar
- 1/2 cup vegan milk
- 2 tbsp. agave
- 1 tsp salt
- 2 tsp vanilla extract

Instructions

1. Preheat oven to 350 F.
2. Mix sugar, milk, brown rice syrup, vanilla extract, and salt in a bowl
3. Add flour to mixing bowl and mix well
4. Dough should be thick enough to need mixing by hand
5. Form small balls from the mixture and place on a lightly oiled cookie sheet
6. Bake for ten minutes
7. Switch the baking sheets on the racks at around the 5 minute mark
8. Take the truffles out of the oven and let them cool before serving

# Chocolate Caramel Truffles

Ingredients

- 1 cup vegan chocolate chips
- 2 cups medjool dates
- 2 tbsp. peanut butter

Instructions

1. Soak dates in warm water for 15 minutes and then drain
2. Pour dates in a food processor and blend until smooth
3. Add the peanut butter to the dates and blend again
4. Scoop out the mixture with a tablespoon and place on a piece of parchment paper
5. Place in freezer for about one hour
6. Melt the vegan chocolate chips in the microwave while the truffles cool
7. Remove truffles from freezer and coat then with the melted chocolate using a spoon
8. Freeze for another 10 minutes before serving

# Chocolate Coconut Balls

Ingredients

Filling

- 1 cup of dried coconut
- 2 tbsp. of maple syrup
- 1/4 cup coconut oil
- 1/8 tsp sea salt
- 1 tsp. of vanilla extract

Coating

- 1/2 cup melted coconut oil
- 2 tsp of maple syrup
- 1/4 cup cacao powder
- 1 pinch sea salt

Instructions

Filling

1. Mix all ingredients in a blender and blend until combined
2. Shape the mixture into small balls and place the coconut balls on a plate lined with baking paper
3. Place in the freezer and prepare the coating

Coating

4. Mix all ingredients in a blender and blend
5. Take the coconut balls out of the freezer and coat them with the chocolate sauce
6. Place them in the refrigerator for 20 minutes

# Chickpea Cookie Dough

Ingredients

- 1 can of chickpeas
- 1/4 cup coconut sugar
- 1/2 cup peanut butter
- 1 tsp vanilla essence
- A handful of dark chocolate chips
- Pinch of salt

Instructions

1. Drain the can of chickpeas
2. Put the chickpeas into a blender
3. Add the rest of the ingredients, except the chocolate chips, and blend
4. Remove from blender and add the dark chocolate chips
5. Mix before serving

# Chapter 6

# 20 Vegan Smoothie Recipes

## Banana and Pineapple

Ingredients

- 3 slices/1 cup diced pineapple
- 2 cups fresh spinach, washed and stems removed
- 1 banana, frozen
- ½ cup fresh orange juice

## Strawberry Banana Smoothie

Ingredients

- 1¼ cups frozen strawberries
- 1 banana, frozen
- ½ cup orange juice

## Blueberry Spinach Pineapple Smoothie

Ingredients

- 1 cup blueberries
- 1 cup pineapple
- 2 cups spinach
- 1 banana, frozen
- ½ cup almond milk

## Banana and Berries Smoothie

Ingredients

- ½ cup raspberries
- ½ cup blueberries
- 1 cup frozen strawberries
- 1 banana
- ½ cup almond milk

## Strawberry Mango Smoothie

Ingredients

- 1 cup strawberries
- ½ frozen banana
- ½ cup almond milk
- 1 cup mango
- ½ frozen banana
- ½ cup milk

## Chocolate Peanut Butter Smoothie

Ingredients

- 1 frozen banana
- 1 cup unsweetened almond milk
- 1 tablespoon runny natural peanut butter – I LOVE Justin's
- 1 tablespoon cocoa/cacao powder

- 1 tablespoon maple syrup

## Turmeric Mango Smoothie

Ingredients

- 1 cup mango
- 1 frozen banana
- ½ teaspoon turmeric
- ½ cup unsweetened almond milk

## Exotic Vegan Smoothie

Ingredients

- 2 Bananas
- 1/2 Papaya
- 1 Mango
- 2 Kiwis
- A dozen strawberries
- 1/2 Cup pineapple (optional)
- One to two cups of cranberry juice to taste

## Vitamin Greens Energy Vegan Smoothie

Ingredients

- Kale
- Mixed Greens
- 2 Carrots

- 2 Apples (core removed)
- 1 Cup Raspberries

## Melon Mixer Vegan Smoothie

Ingredients

- 2 Bananas
- 1/2 Cantaloupe Melon
- 1/4 honeydew melon
- 1/4 Watermelon
- 1 apple

## Peaches and Cream Vegan Smoothie

Ingredients

- 2 Bananas
- 1 Cup of frozen peaches
- 1 Cup Apple Juice

## Vit-C Vegan Smoothie

Ingredients

- 2 Bananas
- 1 Orange
- 2 Kiwis
- A dozen frozen strawberries

- 1/2 Cup of frozen blueberries
- 1-2 Cups of orange juice to taste

## Apple Vegan Smoothie

Ingredients

- 2 Bananas
- 1 green apple
- 1 red apple
- A Dozen frozen strawberries
- Two cups of apple juice to taste

## Sweet and Sour Vegan Smoothie

Ingredients

- 1 Grapefruit
- 1/2 seeded pomegranate
- 1 banana
- 1 teaspoon of mixed seeds

## Peanut Butter Vegan Smoothie

Ingredients

- 1 Cup ice cubes
- 1 Cup soy milk
- 3 to 4 tablespoons of peanut butter
- 1 teaspoon of vanilla extract

- 2 tablespoons maple syrup

## Banana Orange Vegan Smoothie

Ingredients

- 1 Banana
- 1 Cup of soy milk
- 1 orange
- 1/4 cup of orange juice
- 1 teaspoon of raw sugar
- 1/2 cup of ice

## Chocolate Chip Banana Power Smoothie

Ingredients

- 1 1/2 frozen bananas
- 1 C almond milk
- 1/2 C coconut water
- 2 tbsp raw cacao nibs
- 3 tbsp hemp seeds
- 1 tbsp chia seeds
- 1 tbsp almond butter
- 1 tsp maca powder
- 1 pitted medjool date
- 5 ice cubes

## Pineapple Green Tea Smoothie

Ingredients

- 1 cup frozen pineapple
- 3 tbsp oats
- 1 cup almond milk
- 1 tbsp matcha tea powder
- 2 dates, pitted

## Strawberry Spinach Green Smoothie

Ingredients

- 1 1/2 very ripe bananas, peeled, diced and frozen
- 6 oz fresh strawberries, hulled (about 8 - 9 medium)
- 2 mandarin oranges, peeled and halved
- 3 cups packed baby spinach (don't use regular, baby spinach has a milder and sweeter flavor)
- 1 cup cold water
- 1 cup ice

## Banana Oat Breakfast Smoothie

Ingredients

- 1/2 cup non-dairy yogurt
- 1 medium-size ripe banana, frozen
- 1/4 cup almond milk
- 1/3 cup rolled oats

- 1 Tbsp. chia seeds
- ½ tsp. vanilla extract
- Pinch of salt
- 1-2 tsp. maple syrup or honey

# Bonus Chapter

## 10 Workout Vegan Snacks

# Pre-Workout Snacks

**1.** Banana & Peanut Butter: Slice 1 banana and serve with 2 tablespoons all-natural peanut butter.

**2.** Dried fruit: ¼ cup serving of dried berries, apricots, pineapple, raisins or any other dried fruit of your choice

**3.** PB & toast: Spread 1-2 tablespoons of all-natural peanut butter on sprouted grain toast.

**4.** Green Monster Smoothie: 1 cup canned coconut milk, 1 cup spinach leaves, 1 cup kale, 1/2 cup fresh pineapple, 1 frozen banana, 1/2 cup ice cubes, 1/2 cup water. Place all ingredients into a blender and mix until smooth.

**5.** Granola and Milk: ½ cup granola topped with 1 cup of dairy free milk of your choice.

# Post-Workout Snacks

**1.** Banana Ice-Cream: 2 frozen bananas, Almond Milk and 1 scoop protein powder. Place the bananas and protein powder in blender and add a little bit of the milk, and blend together adding more milk as needed.

**2.** Chocolate Milk: Blend 1 cup of almond with 1 Tbsp. of raw cocoa powder and 3 large pitted dates.

**3.** Fruit Cup: Cut and mix to fill one cup: berries, rock melon, banana and orange. Sprinkle 2 TBSP of chia seeds for healthy fats and quality protein.

**4.** Super Energy Booster Smoothie: Place everything in your high speed blender and blend until well combine: 1 tbsp. raw cacao powder, 1 tbsp. chia seeds,1 tbsp. hemp seeds, 1/2 cup coconut milk, 1 cup of almond milk, 1/4 teaspoon cinnamon.

**5.** Carrots, Apples and Hummus: ½ an apple and ½ cup of raw carrots with two spoonfuls of hummus.

# Conclusion

Thank you again for downloading this book!

I hope this book was able to help you switch to plant based diet and gave you a lot of ideas for what you can eat as a vegan.

The next step is to teach what you've learned in this book to the people around you and share with them your new lifestyle.

Finally, if you enjoyed this book, then I'd like to ask you for a favor, would you be kind enough to leave a review for this book on Amazon? It'd be greatly appreciated!

Thank you and good luck!

# Check Out My Other Book

I've written another book on this subject titled 'The Vegan Power: Why Going Vegan Will Save Your Life.' The book offers compelling information on why you should go vegan. It presents information of the diet and lifestyle in general, the benefits of the vegan diet to health, veganism's impact on the environment, and veganism and its influence on emotions and spirituality. Lastly, the book teaches you the steps to shift to veganism and stick to it for the long term. If you'd like to learn more about Veganism and how to live with a Vegan lifestyle, I highly recommend this book.

www.ingramcontent.com/pod-product-compliance
Lightning Source LLC
Chambersburg PA
CBHW071407280526
45787CB00001B/465